The Sex Habits
of Americans

The Sex Habits of Americans

The Inside Story about What Everyone Else Is Doing behind Closed Doors

Amy Winter

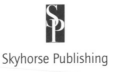

Skyhorse Publishing

Skyhorse Publishing books may be purchased in bulk at special discounts for sales promotion, corporate gifts, fund-raising, or educational purposes. Special editions can also be created to specifications. For details, contact the Special Sales Department, Skyhorse Publishing, 307 West 36th Street, 11th Floor, New York, NY 10018 or info@skyhorsepublishing.com.

Skyhorse® and Skyhorse Publishing® are registered trademarks of Skyhorse Publishing, Inc.®, a Delaware corporation.

Visit our website at www.skyhorsepublishing.com.

10 9 8 7 6 5 4 3 2 1

Library of Congress Cataloging-in-Publication Data is available on file.

ISBN: 978-1-61608-419-6

Printed in China

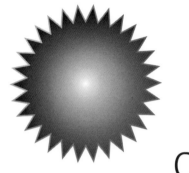

Contents

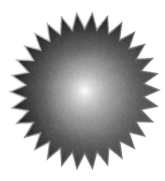

Introduction

You don't want to talk about it or even whisper it, but I'm sure you're thinking about it. In fact, you were probably thinking about it earlier today. It's on billboards, movies, the Internet, and right here in this book. Not that is has to be: Americans are wired for sex. And with a culture as energetic, outgoing, and passionate as ours—we're going to think about it . . . a lot. But with so much sex on the American brain, what about all the things we don't know: the who, what, where, when, why, and how?

. . .

That's where *The Sex Habits of Americans* comes in! There are thousands of books about the American sex drive, and along with various surveys, magazines, and websites, this information has been gathered not only to teach you, but to inform and entertain you. All the answers, details, and numbers have been compiled here to satisfy those curious cravings.

• • •

Nothing seems at once as basic and complicated as sex—it's biology, after all. But what do all those terms really mean? When does a date become "hooking up"? How much sex are Americans having, anyway? What really turns on the other sex? Whether or not you were paying attention in the 8th grade, this book offers a course in Sex Ed., exploring how surprising the 'basics' really are.

• • •

We might be famous for our diversity and tolerance, but what characterizes Americans under the sheets? A romantic might say that eyes are the window into the soul, but nothing reveals real personality like a night in the sack. Rich with varied people and preferences, it turns out that the U.S. is just as colorful, creative, and remarkable in bed as it is in the street. And even though all people may be created equal, not all places are. Where you live might have something to do with whether you were watching TV or getting friendly on the couch last weekend.

. . .

And in the U.S. what people prefer may not only surprise you, but be all around you. This book provides a glimpse into the deep reaches of America's sexual psyche—including your friends, neighbors, and people in the supermarket. There are possibilities everywhere, whether it's a teacher with a double life, a doctor with adventurous tastes, or a neighbor who dreams up an old flame. You can't help but wonder how well you really know America, and then be stunned by the view. It's insight into the private life of a nation, with all its turn ons, anxieties, and anticipations.

• • •

Great research and time went into searching the depths of America's sex habits, and the results were surprising. Interestingly, one gender's perception of the other doesn't always align with reality. They might even agree more than you thought possible! Fantasies take an important place in the sexual psyche, too, and healthy Americans can't help but let their imaginations run wild. It's often the most curious things that will get the American heart to quiver and loins to stir. The sheer amount of fascinating details will suck you in—it's all the emotions and thoughts racing through people before the fall, post-coitus, and *in medias res*. Technique is perhaps the most subjective of topics. On their nights out, men will banter over beers and women will share secrets with each other. But even if your friends don't spare the most sensitive questions, this book doesn't leave out the details on positions, size, and pressure points. Everybody knows what they like best—and Americans can be wildly different. But if you'd rather not share with your friends some of the more intimate pleasures and fears keeping you up at night—you'll find some solace here. The worst mistake during sex? Orgasms (or a lack thereof)? And who might be faking them—and why?

• • •

Sex is important—no point in denying it. You can only gain from considering all those questions that swirl all around it, and this book brings together all the scattered, varied knowledge that we all want to know. Answers to the questions we find impossible to ignore . . . biological, after all. But this is no anatomy textbook—it's meant to provide understanding, advice, and more than a little fun on a topic that's on your mind—several times a day. It's important, curious, and entertaining all at once—simple yet complicated. So what are you waiting for?

· · ·

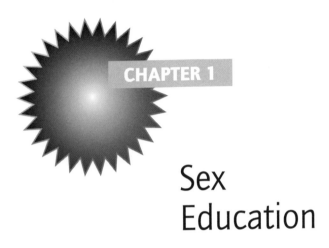

CHAPTER 1

Sex Education

Whether or not your teachers taught you the 'fundamentals' of sex, chances are there were some holes in your education (besides the anatomical ones). And regardless of the how well that formal schooling went, there have always been two sides of the story—one from the teachers and one from growing up. We all learn two vocabularies for the same topic—and in their own way each can be pretty mysterious when you think about it. The technicalities always stay the same, but there's no helpful wisdom from the adults at school, and young people learn from each other—including all the advice, mistakes, jokes and (in)sensible explanations therein. Finally the ultimate teacher, experience, gives us each a subjective lesson on the topic. But this very subjectivity means the lesson is both intense and possibly unreliable. So learning about sex ends up being a lot like putting together a jigsaw puzzle—with pieces from school, peers, and experience. Where to start? Like other

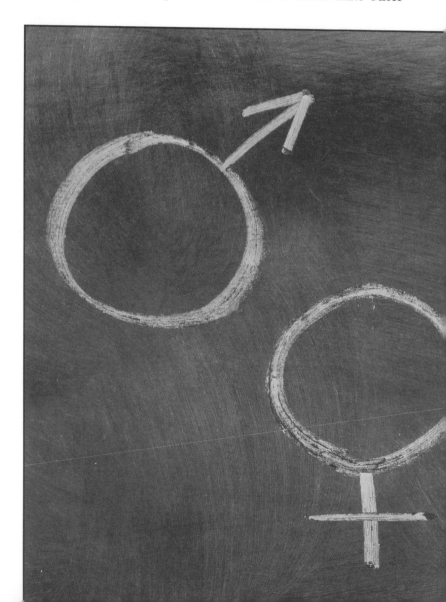

great mysteries of life, the more you learn about sex the more you realize that it's subtle and surprising. There are always puzzle pieces waiting to be found, shuffled, and put together. There's always more to learn.

• • •

This chapter seeks to collapse the various sources of sexual education into a clear framework—the foundation for a sexual reeducation on the habits of Americans. The blueprint for the jigsaw puzzle. It doesn't shy from the technical or the casual, including both the basic statistics and a key to the essential language that we use everyday in modern America. If there have ever been question marks around 'average' or 'safe sex,' look no further. If there have ever been blurry boundaries between 'hooking up' or 'bases,' the definitions are here. If you have any questions, turn the page . . .

• • •

According to a study conducted by Durex condoms, those who reported their parents as the main source of sex and relationship education are 43% more likely to indicate a need to learn more about sex and relationships. Those who rely on teachers, siblings, and nurses to learn about sex are less likely to report a need for more sex education. And those who rely on the Internet to learn about sex are 113% more likely to demonstrate a need for further sex education.

• • •

According to the *New York Times*, sex education curricula in the United States were first developed by Progressive Era reformers like Sears, Roebuck's president, Julius Rosenwald, and Charles Eliot, president of Harvard University from 1869-1909.

• • •

A survey by Harris International shows 83% of Americans believe sexual education should be taught in public schools.

· · ·

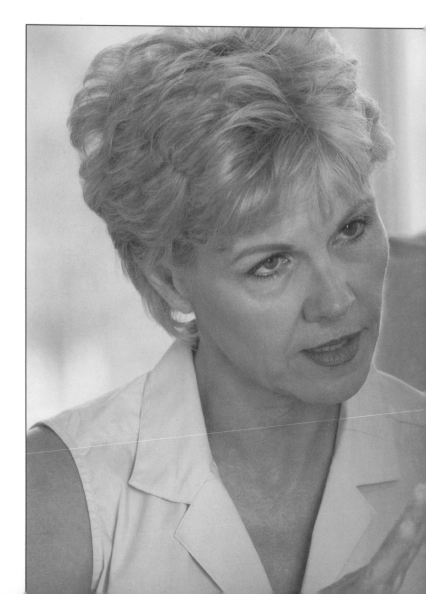

According to a poll conducted by National Public Radio (NPR), 7% of Americans think sex education should not be taught in schools.

. . .

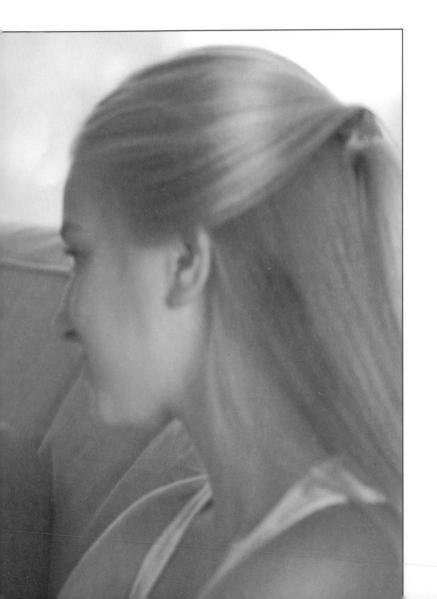

In addition, 74% of American principals polled by NPR say there have been no recent discussions about whether to teach sex ed, and little debate about what kind of sex education should be taught.

• • •

The federal and state governments have spent over $1.5 billion on abstinence-only-until-marriage programs despite evidence that they do not work, according to Advocates for Youth.

• • •

According to NPR, 15% of Americans believe that schools should teach only about abstinence and should not provide information on how to obtain and use condoms and other forms of contraception.

. . .

According to Advocates for Youth, no highly effective sex education is eligible for federal funding because mandates prohibit educating youth about the benefits of condoms and contraception.

. . .

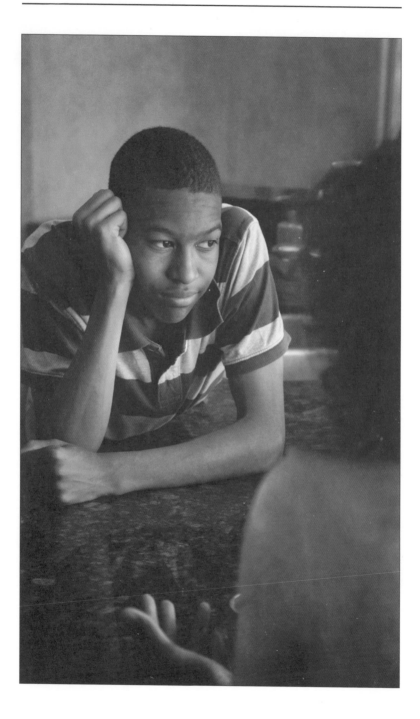

A poll by NPR shows that 30% of public middle schools and high schools teach an abstinence-only curriculum.

• • •

According to the Resource Center for Adolescent Pregnancy Prevention (ReCAPP), only 13% of Americans believe students should be taught an abstinence-only curriculum.

• • •

Another poll from NPR states that 46% of Americans say that the most appropriate approach is one that might be called "abstinence-plus"—schools should teach abstinence as well as condoms and contraception methods.

• • •

But, only 47% of schools (middle and high that teach sex education) teach an abstinence-plus curriculum.

• • •

According to ReCAPP, 99% of Americans believe it is important for young people to have information about STDs, and 94% believe it is appropriate to teach young people about birth control.

• • •

On the other hand, 36% of Americans polled by NPR believe that abstinence is not most important, and sex education in schools should focus on teaching teens how to make responsible decisions.

• • •

In 2007, nearly 90% of students nationwide had never been taught about AIDS or HIV, according to ReCAPP.

. . .

According to NPR, 20% of schools teach that making responsible decisions is more important than abstinence.

. . .

Middle schools are more likely to teach an abstinence-only curriculum than high schools, according to NPR. High schools are more likely than middle schools to teach abstinence-plus. High schools and middle schools were equally likely to teach that abstinence is not the most important thing.

．．．

According to Centers for Disease Control and Prevention (CDC) findings, female teenagers were more likely than male teenagers to talk to their parents about "how to say no to sex," methods of birth control, and where to get birth control.

．．．

In an NPR poll of American parents, 60% think their daughters are very prepared to deal with sexual issues, while only 36% said the same of their sons.

• • •

According to a study conducted by the makers of Durex condoms, kids who reported their parents as the main source of sex and relationships education are 43% more likely to indicate a need to learn more about sex and relationships.

• • •

Fathers are just as likely as mothers to say their daughters are very prepared sexually (60% and 59% those surveyed by NPR, respectively.) However, fathers are much less likely, 23%, to say that their sons are very prepared sexually, while 45% of mothers would say their sons were very prepared.

. . .

In another survey by NPR, 47% percent of parents think girls should wait until they are married to have sexual intercourse, and 44% think boys should wait until they are married.

. . .

But, 89% percent of parents don't think that girls will actually wait that long; 91% feel that way about boys.

• • •

According to the makers of Durex condoms, kids who learn about sex primarily from the Internet are 113% more likely to demonstrate a need for further sex and relationship education.

• • •

Those who relied on a combination of teachers, siblings, and nurses as their primary form of sexual education were least likely to need further education.

. . .

According to NPR, about 19% of American parents think schools should not teach about homosexuality at all.

. . .

The survey further showed that 52% said schools should teach "only what homosexuality is, without discussing whether it is wrong or acceptable," compared with 18% who said schools should teach that homosexuality is wrong, and 8% who said schools should teach that homosexuality is acceptable.

• • •

According to NPR, when asked what concerns them about their 7th–12th-grade children having sexual intercourse, 36% of parents said "that they might have sexual intercourse before they are psychologically and emotionally ready"; 29% said their biggest concern was diseases (23% said HIV/AIDS and 6% said other sexually transmitted diseases); 23% said pregnancy.

• • •

Almost half (48%) of all high school students in the U.S. have had sex, according to Advocates for Youth.

• • •

Advocate for Youth's evaluations of comprehensive sex education programs show that such programs do not lead to earlier first sexual encounters, more sexual encounters, or increase the frequency of sex or the number of sex partners among already sexually active young people.

• • •

Approximately 90% of young men (ages 15–19) had received formal education about birth control or abstinence according to the Guttmacher Institute's study on Young Men's Sexual and Reproductive Health. There were no significant differences between genders.

• • •

Slightly more than half (52%) of young men report that they have talked with a parent about STIs; only 33% have discussed methods of birth control. And, 27% of males had never received information about birth control from either school or parents.

• • •

On average, young males in the United States lose their virginity at age 16.9; females at 17.4, according to the website LiveScience.com. However, aside from sex education, new research shows that genetics may be another factor—traits like impulsivity can be inherited and contribute to a person's willingness to have sex at an earlier age.

. . .

In contrast to the United States, according to *Time Magazine*, Holland has a more comprehensive system of sex education with less sexual stigmatization and teen birth rates that are eight times lower than in the U.S.; U.S. abortion rates are twice as high; U.S. AIDS rate is three times higher than the Dutch. Two-thirds of Dutch parents report allowing their teenage children to have sleepovers with their boyfriend or girlfriend . . . but Americans may just prefer their children learn sooner rather than later to appreciate sex in strange places.

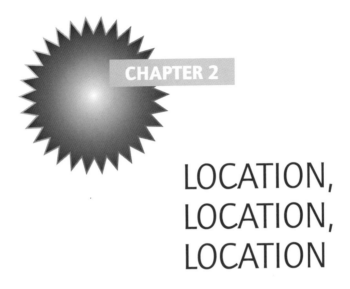

CHAPTER 2

LOCATION, LOCATION, LOCATION

The answer might seem to obvious to ask where are Americans having sex—in their American beds, right? But like everything that has to do with our sexual impulses, it's just not that simple. If you've ever traveled to a new city or coast somewhere along the country, you may have noticed—the people here look, act, speak differently. It's part of what makes us great—travelling up and down the East Coast alone you'll find all sorts of people, looking good, more outgoing, huddling from cold, going to the beach, more conservative or uninhibited ... And it stands to reason that if they're looking, acting and speaking differently from one another, then they're sleeping with one another differently, too. Turns out the facts back up the theory. Cities and regions vary in their habits all around the country—where you live really does affect your sex life!

• • •

And that's only one half of it—Americans have definite preferences as to where they want to be for their intimate moments. Where a man or woman wants to be for sex is intuitively important—sex is as much (and often more) about desire as the physical, and so all those thoughts and emotions tied up in a place can make a big difference when it comes to doing the deed itself. People should have sex in the places they most want to be—and not be wishing they were somewhere else!

• • •

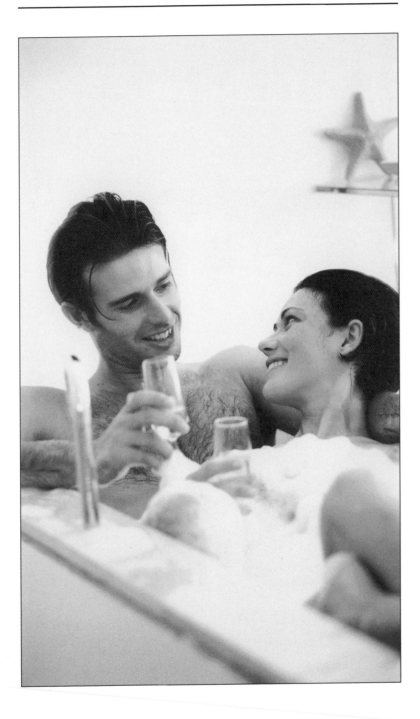

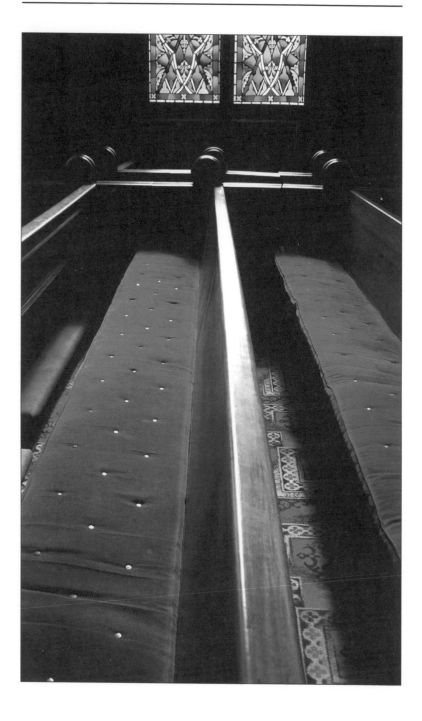

Nearly 47% of American men and almost 43% of American women reported in a *Men's Health* magazine poll that they've had sex in public.

• • •

According to a *Cosmo* magazine survey, the most popular places American adults are having sex outside of their bedrooms are: the shower or bathtub (82% of those surveyed); the car (80%); childhood bedroom (65%); the pool (54%); the woods (49%); the kitchen table (48%); the park (42%); a tent (37%); parents' bedroom (34%); and the laundry room (29%).

• • •

According to ABC news, 57% of Americans say they've had sex in an outdoor or public place.

• • •

The most common place outside of their bed for Americans to have sex is in a car, with 48% of Americans claiming it to be the most exciting venue; followed closely by someone else's bed (33%).

• • •

The riskiest places Americans have reported having sex, according to FOX News are: in a *graveyard*—in Amherst, MA, students often visit the graveyard of Emily Dickinson for hooking up sessions; *nightclubs*—darkened corners and bathroom stalls, along with alcoholic beverages and loud music often provide a perfect setting; in a *raft or canoe*—rocking the boat adds a bit of excitement to the deed; *church pews*—O Lord!; *phone booth*—a nod to the days of yesterday when these were actually used for calls.

. . .

ABC News reports that 12% of Americans are having sex at their workplace, while 1 in 5 indulge in consensual sex with their coworkers.

. . .

The Trojan U.S. Sex Census shows that residents of the Los Angeles metropolitan area are having the most sex per year, averaging 135 times.

. . .

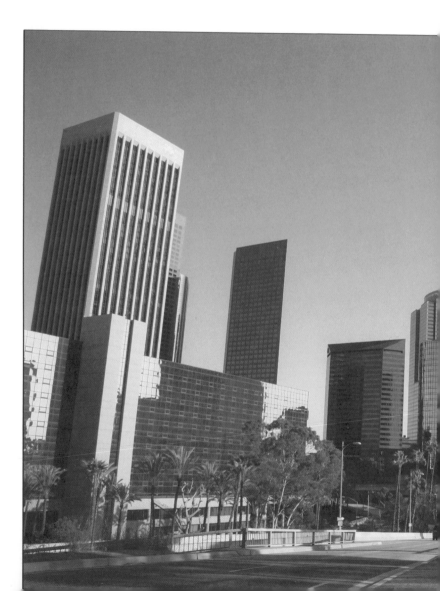

Los Angeles also proves to be the most promiscuous American city with the average number of sexual partners estimated to be 15, according to Mingle2.com. In addition, 75% of Angelenos claim to be sexually satisfied.

• • •

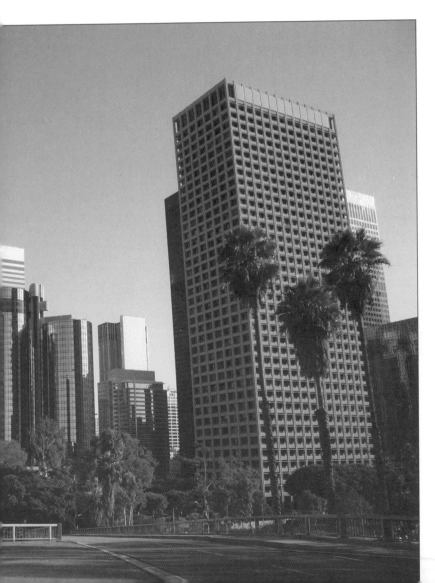

However, the Trojan survey shows with lower levels of sexual frequency, Philadelphians report the highest rates of sexual satisfaction (82%).

· · ·

Regionally, American sexual frequency is highest in the Northeast according to the survey. Americans in the Northeast report having the most sex, averaging 130 times per year (2.5 times per week), compared to the Midwest (125 times per year / 2.4 times per week), West (120 times per year / 2.3 times per week) and South (114 times per year / 2.1 times per week).

· · ·

Other metropolitan centers throughout the country like Houston, TX, report high numbers: 125 times per year, according to the makers of Trojan condoms. Both San Francisco Bay area residents and residents of Mobile, AL, average 12 sexual partners.

• • •

The least promiscuous cities in America are Arcadia, CA; Potomac, MD; Provo, UT; and Sugarland, TX, with averages of 3 sexual partners, according to a Mingle2.com poll.

• • •

According to *SELF* magazine, the city with the healthiest sex lives is Seattle, WA, boasting numerous physicians for women (OB/GYN), 29%; fewer sexually transmitted infections, and 43% fewer deaths from cervical cancer than average. Washington state laws require prescription plans to cover birth control and pharmacies to dispense it, while most other states don't.

. . .

While overall sexual satisfaction in America is high, according to the Trojan U.S. Sex Census, research finds that married couples reported higher satisfaction rates (82% married vs. 71% when single.) Likewise, within every age group from age 18 to over 70, when compared to their peers, people had more sex in marriages than when single.

. . .

Surprisingly, some people in the world are still having sex on beds—inexpensive, mass-produced, easily assembled, Swedish beds. Across the pond, an estimated 10% of all children in Europe are conceived on Ikea beds, according to OMG-Facts.com.

According to research from *Cosmo* magazine, internationally, Australian women are more likely than Americans to be satisfied with their sex lives—27% say they "wouldn't change a thing."

. . .

While Americans, Brits, and Canadians report on average that 20 sexual partners makes a woman a "slut," Australians are less judgmental, claiming the 50th partner is when a woman becomes a "slut" or a man becomes a "man-whore."

· · ·

An estimated 23% of Brits are having sex with their co-workers—about 3% more than the American numbers.

· · ·

Couples in Greece have the most sex in the world, according to RandomHistory.com, approximately 164 times per year. Brazil is a close second at 145 times per year. The global average is 103.

· · ·

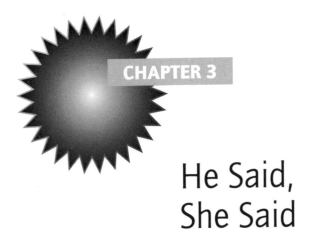

CHAPTER 3

He Said,
She Said

Supposedly, the Great Gender Wars have been raging since Adam and Eve, but peace may be round the corner—or at least more sex! Emotions glower, words let loose, and sparks fly, and before you know it someone's either on the couch or on top of somebody else. The genders often have quite a bit of trouble understanding each other, much less communicating, and plenty of magazines have taken advantage of everybody's confusion. Each side has evolved to think its own way, and even to counter the behavior and feelings of the opposite sex! With even biology telling us

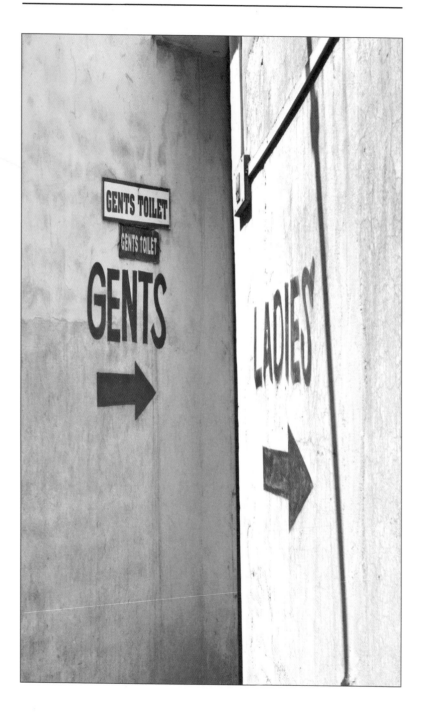

that war and love may not be so different, things tend to get complicated quickly. How to understand the other sex? Or the fire that heats up so fast between them?

. . .

It turns out that the ways men and women understand each other are compelling and curious—signs that though they still battle, they have as many things in common as misunderstandings. It may not surprise you that men's opinions on themselves don't exactly agree with those of women, but it's the 'how' that makes it so interesting. The sexes often want and feel the same things (more sex, usually!). When they don't understand each other, the truth is often a happy surprise, or at least a fascinating glimpse into the way the other side thinks! The 'War' goes on, but both sides are after the same things, and both sides can get them. Whether you read this for a battle plan or you just want to see all the ways we (mis)understand each other—see what they said!

. . .

According to a 2011 *Playboy* readers poll of men and women, 23% of men and 15% of women masturbate at least once a day. According to an identical poll conducted in 1983, 19% of men and 9% of females masturbated as often.

. . .

When asked in a *Men's Health* magazine survey, 46.9% of men report that they think their partner masturbates less than once a month; 32.7% of women think their partner masturbates 2-3 times a week

. . .

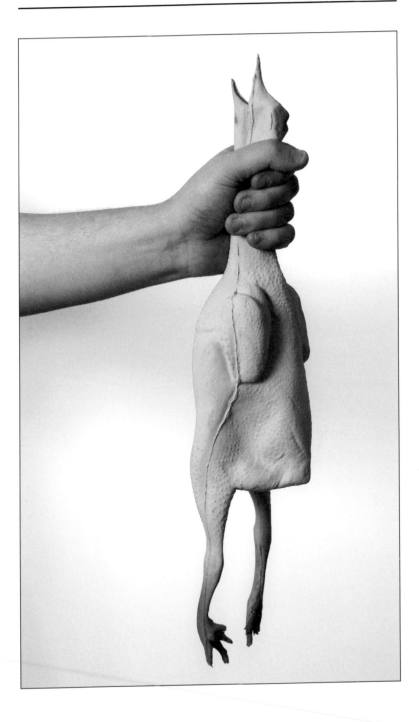

According to research firm Harris Interactive, 31% of American men and 20% of American women have masturbated with someone else.

. . .

A recent poll showed that 44% of men and 37% of women masturbated a few times a week, compared to 31% of men and 19% of women in 1983.

. . .

The poll further showed that 12% of men and 14% of women masturbated once a week and 8% of men and 15% of women masturbate less than once a month.

. . .

Almost 31% of men and 16.4% of women don't think it's okay to ask their partner how many sexual partners they've had, according to a *Men's Health* magazine sex survey.

• • •

Another 5% of males admitted to *Playboy* magazine that they've had sex with more than 100 people.

• • •

An almost identical number, 26.4% of men and 26% of women in a *Men's Health* magazine sex survey, say that the ideal number of sexual partners for their partner to have had is 2-3. Only 2.8% of women and 1.7% of men would be okay if their partner had 51+ sexual partners in their past

• • •

According to Harris Interactive, when asked "How do you personally define sex?" 94% of all respondents agreed that vaginal sex was sex (92% of men and 95% of female); 60% believed oral sex was sex (67% of men and 54% of women); 52% said anal sex counted (58% of men and 47% of women). Another 4% choose the option "other" when defining sex.

. . .

According to *Men's Health*, 41.8% of men haven't asked how many partners their current partner has had; 68.1% of women have asked.

. . .

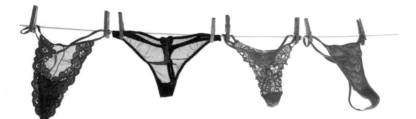

Approximately 36% of men and 32% of women surveyed by *Playboy* had 1-5 sex partners. Almost 20 years prior, 30% of men and 37% of women had the same amount of sex partners.

. . .

The survey also showed that 41% of men and 55% of women had 6-25 sex partners and 10% of men and 9% of women had more than 51 sexual partners.

. . .

According to *Men's Health* magazine, 37.5% of men and 31.6% of women have lied about how many sexual partners they've had, the majority fudging the number by 1 or 2.

• • •

According to Harris Interactive, 57% of men didn't know the first and last names of all the people they've had sex with; 73% of women did.

• • •

Our 36th President of the United States, Lyndon B. Johnson, is alleged to have nicknamed his penis "Jumbo." He was supposedly also fond of waving his penis around, according to Cracked.com. Rumor has it that in competing with JFK's legacy, Johnson was a serial philanderer—soliciting sex from many of his secretaries and aides and using the Secret Service to keep word of his exploits from his wife.

According to *Men's Health* magazine, a majority of both men and women, nearly 65%, don't count past oral sex partners as sex partners.

• • •

In a *Playboy* reader poll, 79% of men and 85% of women reported to have talked dirty during sex, a large increase from the 1983 version of the poll where only 40% of men and 47% of women did the same.

• • •

Men are more likely to have cheated, according to ABC News, much more likely to fantasize about cheating, and twice as likely as women to say it's okay to have casual sex without a committed emotional relationship.

• • •

In a survey of Americans conducted by Harris Interactive, 18% of men and 14% of females cheated while in a supposedly monogamous relationship.

• • •

According to OMG-Facts.com, men who are risk takers are more likely to cheat, whereas women are more likely to cheat when they are dissatisfied with their current relationships or if they feel sexually incompatible with their partners.

• • •

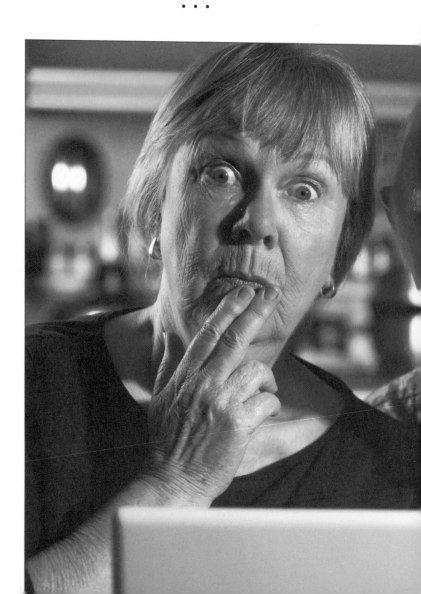

Also, 23% of men and 19% of women reported to *Playboy* that they've cheated on a spouse, a drop from the 36% of men and 34% of women who cheated in 1983.

. . .

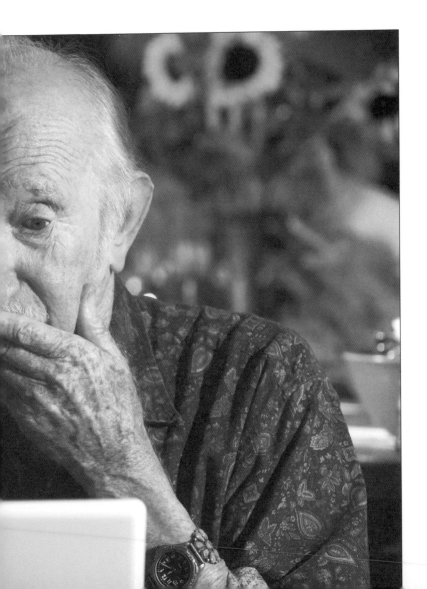

According to Harris Interactive, 39% of men and 23% of women think they can forgive a partner who cheats. But, 34% of men and 39% of women weren't sure; 39% of men and 38% of women definitely wouldn't be able to forgive.

. . .

In another poll by *Men's Health* magazine, 30.4% of men and 19.7% of women think that oral sex technique is most important for pleasing a woman

. . .

When researchers for Harris Interactive asked, "How often do you perform oral sex on your partner?" 19% of men and 11% of women said every time they have sex; 28% of men and 18% of women said most times; 31% of men and 38% of women said occasionally; 17% of men and 26% of women claimed never.

• • •

According to *Slate*, 88% of women say they've received oral sex from a man, and 72% say they've received it in the last year. The men's numbers corroborate: 86% said they've given it; 91% of men say they've received oral sex

• • •

Of those who read *Playboy*, 78% of men and 79% of women have watched porn. Only 38% of men and 42% of women watched porn in 1983.

• • •

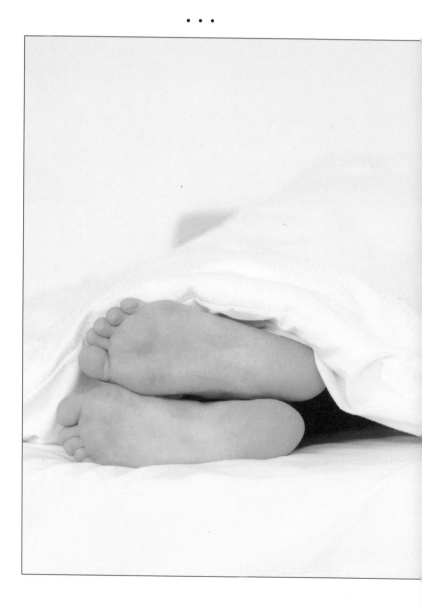

Also, 57.3% of men and 47.6% of women have had sex while watching pornography according to *Men's Health* magazine.

. . .

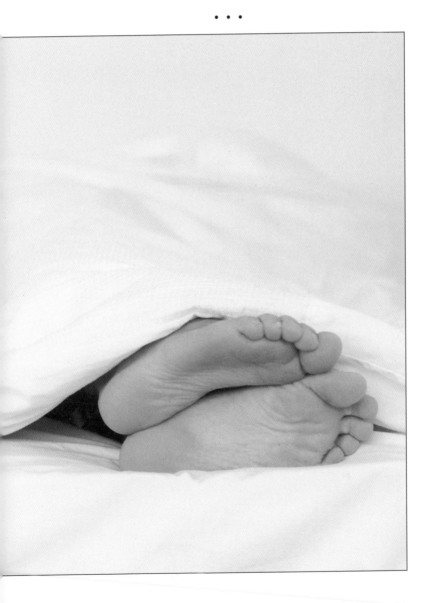

According to Harris Interactive, 55% of men would like more sex. Only 34% of women feel the same, while 5% of women would like less.

• • •

In a *Men's Health* magazine sex survey, when men and women were asked "How often do you want sex?" 34.8% of men and 35.1% of women said two or three times a week; 30% of men and 26.3% of women said once a day; 25% of both men and women want sex several times a day; 3.81% of men and 6.3% of women want sex once a week; and 6.1% of men and 6.8% of women wanted sex less than once a week.

• • •

Sex can increase estrogen levels for women, which protects against osteoporosis, Alzheimer's and endometriosis, according to SmashingLists.com.

• • •

For men, evidence suggests that having sex weekly can lower risk of heart disease by 30%, stroke by 50%, and diabetes by 40%, according to RandomHistory.com. An active sex life can lead to men living past 80 years.

• • •

According to *Men's Health* magazine, 53.7% of men and 29.1% of women say they would never turn down sex.

• • •

Forty-five percent of all *Playboy* readers, male and female, admit to having had sex with more than one person in the course of one day.

. . .

According to Harris Interactive, 38% of men and 14% of women admit to sleeping with two people within 24 hours.

. . .

Researchers have found that having sex twice or more a week reduced the risk of fatal heart attack by half for men, according to WebMD's assessment of the health benefits of sex.

· · ·

A *Men's Health* survey reported that 66.3% of men want their partner to initiate sex more often; 35.2% of women feel the same. Also, 1.25% of men and 6.2% of women want their partners to initiate sex less often.

· · ·

According to WebMD, women who have sex at least once a week have more regular menstrual cycles than those who have sex less frequently. Sex generally helps promote fertility in women by regulating their menstrual patterns.

• • •

According to Harris Interactive, 24% of men and 13% of women never tell their partners before sex that they've been diagnosed with an STD.

• • •

According to *Cosmo* magazine, amongst the various reasons men have for being taken out of the mood for sex, their partner's self-image issues rank the highest.

. . .

According to the *Men's Health* sex survey, 15.6% of women claimed to be much more likely to turn down sex because they need more time to warm up. Other reasons women were more likely to turn down sex include: their partner taking too long to orgasm, needing an emotional connection, or their partner wants too much sex.

. . .

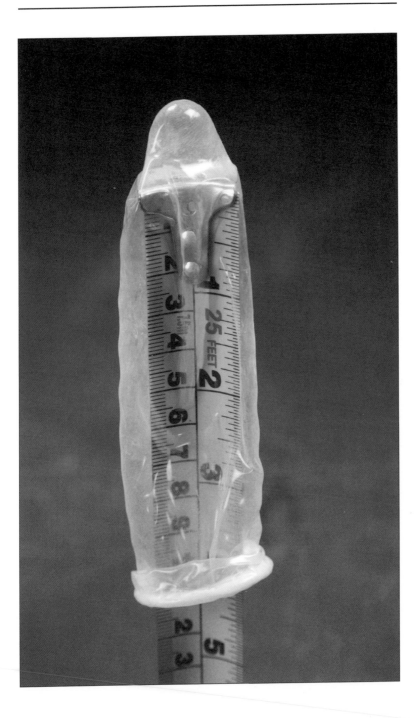

Approximately 30% of men and 32% of women shave their pubic hair, according to Harris Interactive.

• • •

Women were more likely (67.4% of those surveyed by *Men's Health* magazine) to prefer their own pubic area to be completely bald or their pubic hair kept very short. But, 32.3% of men prefer their partner's pubic hair to be shaved or waxed into shapes.

• • •

Nearly 50% of men would groom their pubic region in any way that turns their partner on; 38% of women feel the same.

. . .

Forty percent of women reported to *Cosmo* magazine that their partners were not very or never romantic, while 75% of men claim they are, consistently.

. . .

According to *Men's Health* magazine, men were more likely than women to turn down sex if their partner wanted too much foreplay.

. . .

According to Harris Interactive, 14% of women had to wait a year or more after losing their virginity before having sex again. But only 9% of men waited as long.

. . .

Almost 45% of women would describe their most recent sex partner's penis as about average; 32.3% of women would describe it as "about right." Almost 60% of men would describe their penis as average, according to *Men's Health* magazine.

• • •

According to *Cosmo* magazine, 44% of women said that they're perfectly happy with their breast size. But 52% men want a bigger penis: 30% said it would make themselves feel better and 22% said it would primarily be to better satisfy their partner.

• • •

The ideal girth for an erect penis is the diameter of a D-size battery, according to 74% of men surveyed by *Men's Health* magazine, and 64% of women. 38.3% of men and 34.8% of women consider the ideal length for an erect penis to be 7 inches. Both men and women agreed that the least ideal length for a penis is 1-3 inches.

. . .

Less than 25% of women told *Cosmo* that their partner should always pick up the bill and 40% of women think they should split the bill . . . but the same survey revealed nearly 50% of women believe that splitting the bill can hurt the romance. But, 80% of men think they should just pay for the bill each time.

. . .

Twenty-seven percent of men and 23.4% of women consider a romantic dinner out as the sort of date to most likely put them in the mood for sex, according to *Men's Health* magazine. Slightly more than 26% of men and 28.7% of women would rather have a quiet night at home to put them in the mood for sex.

• • •

According to *Men's Health* magazine, women were more likely than men to be turned on by a date that included dancing, going to a sporting event, or shopping.

• • •

Sex can help prevent breast cancer for women who have never given birth, according to new studies (Smashing-Lists.com).

· · ·

Men who had five or more orgasms weekly while in their 20s reduced their risk of getting prostate cancer by a third, according to WebMd

· · ·

Forty-four percent of men had sex with someone within six hours of meeting them, according to Harris Interactive's survey of Americans; 17% of women have had the same experience.

• • •

Women (19%) reported to *Men's Health* magazine that they were more likely to have sex with a new partner for the first time after several months of dating but want to wait until they're in a committed relationship. Men were most likely to have sex with a new partner after a month of dating (14%) but want to as soon as they get the okay.

• • •

Almost 22% of women tell *Men's Health* that they have sex whenever they want, even on a first date.

• • •

Research cited by WebMD supports a link between partner hugs and lower blood pressure in women in and out of bed.

• • •

Nearly 35% of men find the butt to be most sexy part of women, according to *Men's Health* magazine. But, 23% of men are turned on the most by the chest of a woman. Almost 20% women are turned on most by a man's face. Women are least attracted to a man's legs.

• • •

Forty-two percent of women think that their chest is the most attractive part of their body to the opposite sex, while 26.9% of men believe that their face is the most attractive part of their body to the opposite sex.

• • •

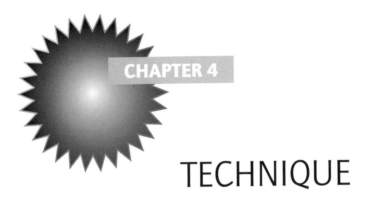

CHAPTER 4

TECHNIQUE

People think of sex like a fine wine: it gets better with age. The simile ends just about there, though, because it'll never improve if you keep your sex life locked in a dark cellar to gather dust. No, all kinds of factors affect whether it's the best night of your lives, leaving you blissfully stunned— or whether it's an awkward encounter that has parties avoiding eye contact and trying to forget the whole thing.

• • •

What makes a difference is knowledge and practice—this chapter can provide the former, you'll have to manage the latter in your private time. But no matter what, you will want to consider the details in the following pages, especially since they cover all the factors that matter most: position, size, motion, duration—all these and more. All of these variables are part of what can make sex so good (or bad), and they're impossible to ignore. Without experience, sex will never get better—but you've got to know what to practice!

• • •

A Polish anthropologist by the name of Bronislaw Malinowski claims the phrase "missionary position" was first coined by indigenous people of the South Pacific after arriving Christian missionaries showed shock and disbelief that the people of the South Pacific had sex in various positions (RandomHistory.com).

• • •

According to a survey conducted by the makers of Trojan condoms, men's favorite sex positions are missionary (27%), followed by doggy style (24%); females report missionary (45%) and reverse missionary (13%) as their top sex positions.

• • •

The favorite sex positions of men surveyed by *Cosmo* magazine include: girl-on-top (28% of men reported), doggie-style (16%), doggie-style with her bent over the bed or couch (16%), missionary with her legs on my shoulders (16%).

• • •

The average sex session lasts from three to ten minutes, according to *Psychology Today*.

• • •

According to Cosmo magazine, 34% of men say 45 minutes is an ideal length of time for a sex session. Another 30% of men think 30 minutes is the ideal amount of time.

• • •

According to WebMD, during just 30 minutes of sex, between 85–200 calories will be burned.

• • •

According to a *Men's Health* sex survey, 49.3% of women want sex to last 5–20 minutes longer on average.

• • •

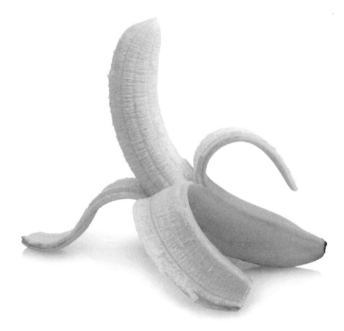

Cosmo magazine reports that 64% of men want to have a quickie (a 10-minute session) 1 to 3 times a week.

• • •

According to LoveLetterBox.com, 25% of all penises bend in some direction.

• • •

For women, doing pelvic floor muscle exercises—Kegel exercises—will lead to more pleasure as well as help to minimize the risk of incontinence later in life, according to WebMD.

• • •

According to ABC News, men are twice as likely as women to sleep naked, and more than half of women surveyed prefer to have sex with the lights off compared to only 27% of men.

• • •

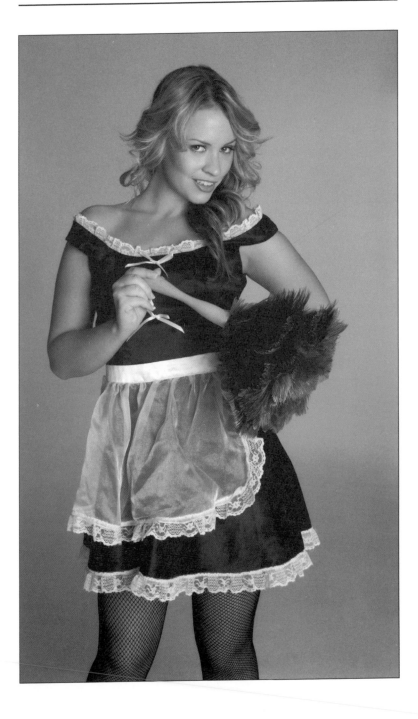

Almost 30% of men reported to *Cosmo* magazine that when their partner refuses to let them see her with the lights on, it ruins the mood; 28% of men reported that when their partner asks if she looks fat, it ruins the mood; and 27% of men reported that when their partner puts down her body/sex skills, it ruins the mood.

• • •

According to a *Men's Health* magazine survey, 55.5% of women say that to please them thrusting technique is most important. On the other hand, 9.2% of women think duration is the most important.

• • •

According to *Cosmo*, 49% of men say the best way for a woman to make sex with a condom more enjoyable is to contract her PC muscles during the act or do positions that create extra friction.

• • •

According to Askmen.com, most women enjoy being on top during sex because it makes them feel like they're in charge but suggest that men not take this as an opportunity to simply "sit back and enjoy the scenery."

• • •

Two-thirds of sexually active Americans report that they've worn "something sexy" to enhance their sex lives, according to an ABC News sex survey

. . .

According to a *Men's Health*'s sex survey, a majority of both men (96%) and women (97.3%) preferred lingerie to be either racy or elegant instead of trashy.

. . .

Sixty-seven percent of men polled by *Cosmo* are most attracted to the girl-next-door-look (ponytail, natural makeup, casual-but-cute outfit, approachable smile). Slightly more than 70% of men claimed a great smile makes them notice a girl the most and 42% of men think women do not play up their legs enough. Only 9% were attracted to the ice queen look (chic hair and makeup, stylish clothes that look expensive, cool vibe).

• • •

Almost 61% of men in a *Men's Health* survey think their partner isn't as adventurous as they'd like while 69.4% of women are satisfied with how adventurous their partner is.

• • •

Sixty-one percent of men surveyed by *Cosmo* prefer a woman to be adventurous and willing to try anything (in and out of bed).

• • •

More than 80% of women 55–64 say they're sexually confident and 62% say they have a good sense of what satisfies them sexually, according to Match.com. The numbers are much lower for younger Americans.

• • •

In a *Men's Health* sex survey, when asked what would get them to be more sexually experimental, 32.6% of women wanted their partner to show how much he respects her and 66% of women said they were more likely to be adventurous with their partner after they've built a trusting relationship with him.

• • •

Almost 60% of men surveyed by *Cosmo* magazine consider "I want you so bad" to be the best thing a girl can say when they first see each other in the nude.

• • •

Almost 45% of men surveyed by *Men's Health* magazine said they're always willing to be sexually adventurous.

• • •

When *Cosmo* asked, "What seduction technique do girls think is sexy but doesn't do anything for you?" 40% of men responded "sucking on my nipples." Nearly 30% of men responded that when their partner gets naked, then says he can't touch her right away, didn't do anything for them. On the other hand, 32% of men think everything their partner does is sexy.

• • •

Eighty-two percent of women have had at least one casual sex partner, according to a recent *SELF* magazine survey; 63% of them say they felt 'great' or 'fine' afterwards. A majority of women polled have had between 1 and 5 casual sex partners, but 5% have had more than 20.

• • •

According to a Trojan sex survey, more than 70% of Americans define hooking up as having sex with someone outside of a relationship, with 40% of women saying they were against hooking up compared to 22% of men.

• • •

According to *Women's Health*, during the college years and a woman's early thirties are the times with the highest number of sexual partners.

• • •

According to the Centers for Disease Control and Prevention (CDC), from a study of 62,000 American women aged 15–44, 22% had one sex partner, 11% had two, and 32% had between three and six. But, 8% had upwards of 15.

• • •

Only 3% of men surveyed by *Cosmo* would want sex to be crazy and experimental all the time but 52% would enjoy that sometimes.

· · ·

Fifty-five percent of women and 50% of men report that they're aroused by being bitten, according to an Indiana University study.

· · ·

Almost 80% of men would love if a woman ambushed them with sex when they least expected it, according to *Cosmo* magazine.

• • •

Nearly 23% of women polled by *Men's Health* magazine say that the worst mistake men make during oral sex is being too rough. Yet, 8.5% of men say their women are often too gentle during oral sex.

. . .

When asked by *Cosmo* magazine what move they would prefer a girl not do during their first time, 65% of men said "touch my back door." The next most popular answers were: using a toy such as a vibrator (48%); tying me up (45%); blindfolding me (41%); and spanking me (39%).

. . .

Men's Health found that 35.9% of men and 28.8% of women think they give more oral sex than they receive and would want it to be more even. On the other hand, 14.1% of men and 21.1% of women say they receive more and like it that way.

• • •

Time magazine found that 14% of men ages 40–49 and 15% of men ages 50–59 reported ever having received oral sex from another man in their lifetimes.

• • •

According to the National Survey of Sexual Health and Behavior, 7% of adult women and 8% of men identify as gay, lesbian, or bisexual. However, the portion of individuals in the U.S. who have had same-gender sexual experiences is much higher.

· · ·

According to *Time* magazine, about 11% of men ages 20 to 24 say they've ever received anal sex in their lives; for men in their 40s and 50s, that figure levels off at about 9%. Among adult women ages 18–29, the rate of ever giving oral sex to another woman ranges from about 8% to 14% and the rate of receiving oral sex ranges from about 8% to 17%.

· · ·

The Gräfenberg Spot, or G-spot, is named after Dr. Ernest Gräfenberg who in 1950 found that stimulation of a particular area in the vagina could trigger powerful orgasms, female ejaculation, and arousal, a find that has confounded many amateur "researchers" since. More recently, according to the *Journal of Sexual Medicine*, ultrasounds show that the clitoris may really be a "clitoral complex" extending along the sides of the vulva, which scientists say may explain why exterior stimulation can be so arousing.

The spoon position, according to AskMen.com, has the advantage of allowing the man to reach around and stimulate the clitoris while penetrating from behind her.

· · ·

Forty-one percent of men surveyed by *Cosmo* want a woman to lead them to her hot spots to signify that she wants to continue being pleasured.

· · ·

Almost 48% of women claim in a survey done by *Men's Health*, the worst mistake that their partner makes is not providing enough foreplay and rushing into sex. Also, 43.9% of men say that their partner doesn't communicate enough.

• • •

Forty-six percent of men surveyed by *Cosmo* described their favorite kind of sex as "playful and energetic." Only 11% described "soft and romantic" as their favorite kind.

• • •

Askmen.com suggests a woman position herself on a surface level to a man's waist as he stands and penetrates, claiming that orgasm is, on average, relatively quick to achieve for the man as well as significantly enjoyable for the woman.

• • •

According to *Cosmo*, 29% of men consider a woman lightly touching their penis to be the best thing she can do post-orgasm.

• • •

Research from the University of Central Lancashire, suggests that the moans and sounds a woman makes during intercourse may not correlate as much to her own pleasure and orgasm, but rather come from her partner's orgasm or her attempts to incite one.

• • •

When asked by *Cosmo*, 41% of men claim hearing their partner moan would be their choice for their only sexual experience for the rest of their lives; 1% said getting their butts slapped.

• • •

Half the men surveyed would want their partner to touch herself while they are having sex. Only 5% would want their partner to not touch herself at all.

• • •

Slightly more than half of women polled by *SELF* magazine said their goal in having a casual fling is to have a good time, fun. Wanting to get out of a relationship was another reason.

• • •

Couples who had sex earliest in their relationship had the worst relationship outcomes according to LiveScience.com.

• • •

Americans are more likely to have sex late at night and generally have no preference as to whether it is a weekend or weekday according to ABC. However 22% prefer the weekend.

• • •

On average, most Americans have sex at 10:34 p.m. on Saturday night according to LoveLetterBox.com.

. . .

The average American adult has sex 56.9 times each year, according to Sloshspot.com. American men have on average 20.8 sexual partners; 6.3 for women. Also, 56% of men and 30% of women have had 5 or more partners in their lifetime.

. . .

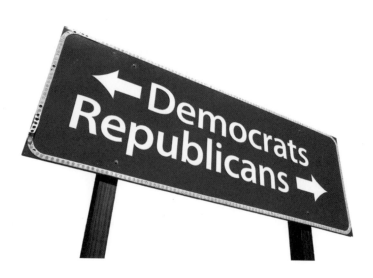

ABC News claims that Republicans are around 10% more likely than their Democrat counterparts to be very satisfied with their marriages and sex lives and to wear something sexy to spice things up; and less likely to admit they've cheated.

• • •

According to the dating site Mingle2.com, fans of golf have the most sexual partners of all other sports fans, averaging 10 in their lifetime. Soccer fans average the least, 6.

• • •

Weekly churchgoers have half as many lifetime sex partners as those Americans that do not attend church weekly according to ABC News.

Some of the sexual bloopers that Match.com members have experienced: falling while being on top during sex and crashing onto his forehead; sex against a hotel room door leading to a broken door and nudity in the hallway; an impromptu threesome with a clawing cat; profuse sweat and stinging eyes.

• • •

Medication, according to *Good Housekeeping* magazine, may cause sexual dysfunction, especially blood pressure and antidepressant drugs. Other culprits include allergy medication and oral contraceptives.

. . .

CNN reports that 3 to 5 Americans per 100,000 are afflicted with transient global amnesia due to sex. Those in their 50s and 60s are most susceptible, and researchers aren't sure what causes it or why patients remain otherwise alert during episodes.

. . .

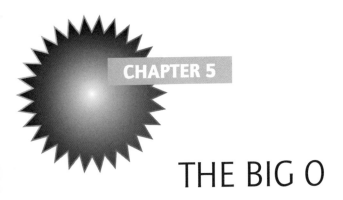

THE BIG O

It can spark hundreds of endorphins, send shudders down your spine, and leave you gasping for breath. It's the satisfaction that everybody craves—fulfillment, release, and blissful exhaustion. It feels good, and it is good! But the best things are rarely simple or easy, and orgasms are no exception.

• • •

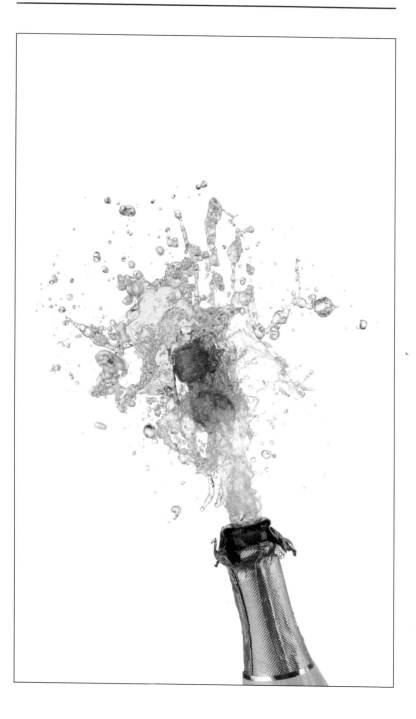

For many Americans, orgasms are far more elusive and difficult than they'd like. Just like technique, they are the product of various factors: physical, mental, emotional, environmental. An individual's preferences in these variables are extremely important, along with their relationship (or lack thereof) with their partner and a moment's circumstances.

. . .

This is not to say that Americans aren't being satisfied in bed. On the contrary, many know their favorite ways of reaching that climax, and have made it loud and clear to their partner as to what works (and communication of all kinds, especially this kind, is heartily encouraged). Though what's loud isn't always an indication of orgasm—anyone's capable of faking it. Who are the actors among us, you might ask? How often? It's all in the following pages, along with the only sure-fire prevention for your partner faking it: the how, when, and why of giving and receiving a real, inimitable orgasm.

. . .

Over a decade ago, 25% of American women reported reaching orgasm as a result of vaginal intercourse. Recently, this has risen to around 45%. In contrast, more than 80% of women report experiencing orgasm through oral sex (RandomHistory.com).

• • •

According to a *Playboy* magazine survey, 54% of American men and 17% of American women reported that they always orgasm during sex. An identical 34% reported that they "usually" orgasm during sex, while 3% of men and 15% of women claimed to rarely orgasm. Only 1% of men and 7% of women surveyed said they never orgasm during sex.

• • •

Almost 76% of men and just 26.8% of women were more likely to reach orgasm from vaginal sex according to a *Men's Health* survey. However, 28.1% of women say they were more likely to reach orgasm by clitoral stimulation.

• • •

A *SELF* magazine sex survey reports that 74% of women have a harder time reaching orgasm when they're with a non-romantic partner. Still, their research shows that women have an easier time getting aroused with a casual partner, even though orgasm itself can be elusive.

• • •

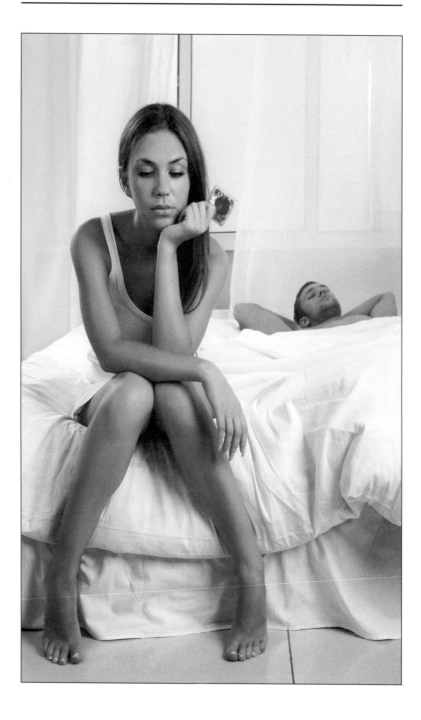

Almost 23% of women surveyed by *Men's Health* said they are most likely to orgasm via direct clitoral stimulation by either themselves or a sex toy. Also, 20.7% of women are most likely to reach orgasm via oral sex.

. . .

According to *Women's Health* magazine, scientists have found that pomegranates are rich in polyphenols, antioxidants that allow blood to flow through veins—contributing to more enjoyable sex.

. . .

Healthy levels of zinc will also contribute to a healthy sex drive and support good sexual function.

• • •

The Kinsey Institute reports that women who use a hormonal contraceptive plus condoms were generally more sexually satisfied. It follows then that when women are less worried about pregnancy and STIs, they can relax and enjoy themselves more.

• • •

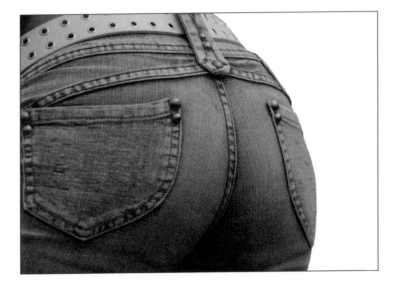

Men were more likely to reach orgasm through their own manual stimulation than through manual stimulation by their female partners according to a *Men's Health* survey.

· · ·

According to a *Prevention* magazine sex survey, low libido is the most common sexual complaint among women of all ages with nearly 40% of women being afflicted at some point in their lives.

· · ·

Nearly 12% of women in the U.S. have never experienced an orgasm. Marilyn Monroe, an international sex symbol, reportedly never experienced an orgasm with any of her famous lovers (RandomHistory.com).

• • •

According to the Kinsey Institute, women are much more likely to be nearly always or always orgasmic when masturbating alone than with another sexual partner. However, among women currently in a relationship, 62% report that they are very satisfied with the frequency/consistency of orgasm.

• • •

According to *Slate* magazine, among women who had vaginal sex in their last sexual encounter, 65% claim to have reached orgasm. Among those who received oral sex, it was 81%. Among those who had anal sex, it was 94%.

. . .

Some theories offered by *Slate* for the correlation between anal sex and orgasms in women include: anal sex directly causes orgasms; orgasms increase a women's willingness to try anal sex; women who orgasm easily are more likely to try anal; love, trust, self-assurance, and comfort cause both orgasms and anal; anal includes manual vaginal stimulation that causes orgasms; masculine assertiveness causes orgasms and anal sex; lastly, pornography possibly increases the prevalence of anal and skews the data.

An identical amount of men as women (48%) claim to have faked an orgasm at least once in their lives (RandomHistory.com).

• • •

According to WebMD, having orgasms increases levels of oxytocin, a hormone that helps us build bonds and trust and increases endorphins. Higher oxytocin levels are also linked with feelings of generosity, relieving pain, and promoting better sleep.

• • •

According to SmashingLists.com, every time you orgasm, the hormone DHEA (dehydroepiandrosterone) increases, leading to a boost in immune system function. DHEA can also repair tissue, improve cognition, keep your skin healthy and work as an antidepressant . . . all of which contribute to a longer, happier life.

. . .

A study from the State University of New York shows that women were less depressed when exposed directly to semen.

. . .

Almost 23% of women are prevented from reaching orgasm because of being distracted according, to *Men's
Health* magazine. 47% of men claim to never have a prob-
lem.

• • •

WebMD reports that premature ejaculation is the most
common form of sexual dysfunction in younger men and
its prevalence is around 20% to 30% in men of all ages.

• • •

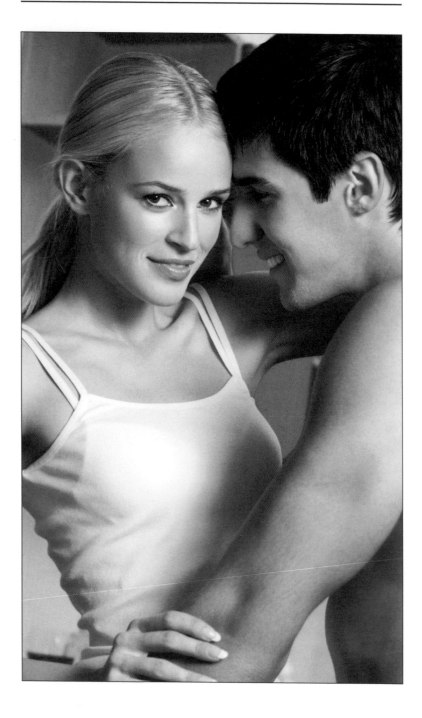

A study in *The Journal of Sexual Medicine* found a median IELT ("intravaginal ejaculatory latency time"/ measure of average ejaculation time for men after penetration) of 5.4 minutes.

. . .

In a survey conducted by *Men's Health* magazine, when asked "Has your partner ever faked an orgasm?" 59.7% of men and 92.9% of women responded "No." (40.3% of men and 7.1% of women replied "Yes.")

. . .

When asked "Have you ever faked an orgasm?" by *Men's Health* magazine, 71.8% of men surveyed and 34.9% responded "No." On the other hand, 28.3% of men and 65.1% of women responded "Yes."

• • •

According to RandomHistory.com, the record for most female orgasms is 134 in one hour.

• • •

According to ABC News, blondes are a little less likely than other women to always have an orgasm, and a little more likely to have faked it.

• • •

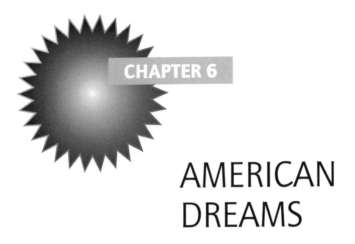

CHAPTER 6

AMERICAN DREAMS

Since the first settlers came to this land, Americans have dreamt big, and done everything in their power to make those dreams happen. Dreams of a brighter future, a wild beauty, and the pursuit of happiness define our national culture. Whether you want a family, passion, or happiness in its many forms—sex is inseparable from the American Dream. The pilgrims may have been Puritans, but modern America's full of their dreams and many more (and the pilgrims had their kid somehow . . . missionary, perhaps?).

· · ·

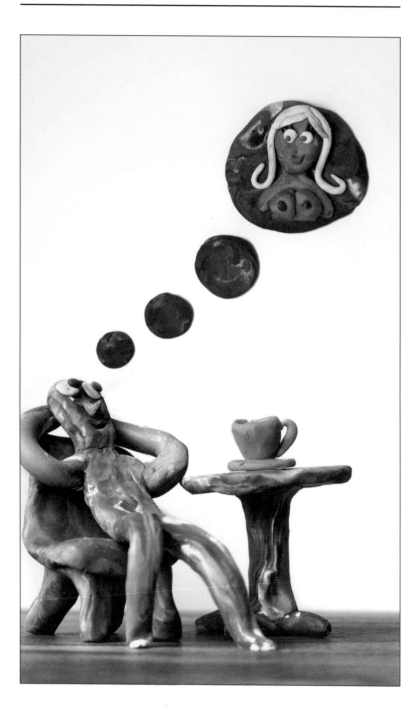

Modern Americans have all the fantasies of their predecessors and a whole set of new ones. It's fascinating to look at whom Americans want to be with, when (and how). Both men and women are fantasizing far more often than you'd think, and not only are the details of the 'gender divide' captivating, but they're rarely what you'd expect. Fantasizing about sex turns out to be a generally healthy habit of Americans; sometimes it's when they act on it that things go poorly. When a relationship moves to quickly or is founded on infidelity—fantasies made reality in the wrong ways—it rarely develops well. But in general, Americans have excelled at balancing the dreams, ambitions, and reality—and the curious details of their fantasies are just as varied and important.

· · ·

A *Cosmos* magazine study found that men and women are equally likely to dream about sex. But while women's fantasies tended to focus on celebrities and past lovers, men tend to visualize themselves making love to multiple partners in public settings, and 90% of men's sex dreams involved women initiating sex.

• • •

Another study from LiveScience.com found that men's dream's feature more reference to sexual activity and intercourse, while women's dreams feature more kissing and less sexually explicit fantasies about other dream characters. The women in this study also had more nightmares.

. . .

A Kinsey Institute study claims that women's fantasies tend to be more emotional and romantic. Men's fantasies mention a partner's sexual desire and pleasure more often than in women's fantasies. American women more often fantasize about taking a passive role or being dominated while men more often fantasize about taking a dominant role, doing something sexual to their partner, according to the Kinsey Institute.

. . .

In a *Men's Health* sex survey, when asked "Why do you fantasize (during sex)?" 46.3% of men and 35.1% of women responded "images just pop into my head."

. . .

But, 43.7% of men and 58% of women answered "it helps me get turned on."

. . .

Only 6.5% of men and 4.5% of women answered "I'm bored."

. . .

But, 3.6% of men and 2% of women answered "to focus on something besides my partner."

. . .

Slightly more than half of men reported to the Kinsey Institute that they think about sex everyday or several times a day, 43% a few times per month or a few times per week, and 4% less than once a month. Nineteen percent of women told researchers they think about sex everyday or several times a day, 67% said a few times per month or a few times per week, and 14% reported thinking about sex less than once a month.

• • •

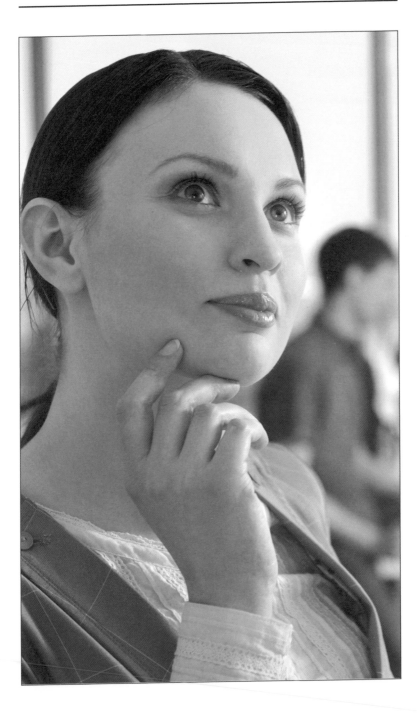

According to a *Men's Health* magazine sex survey, when asked "Do you fantasize?" 43.3% of male and 41% of female respondents answered "yes, but only during masturbation."

. . .

Slightly more than 41% of men and 22.5% of women replied "yes, during sex and masturbation."

. . .

Slightly more than 9% of men and 27.4% of women didn't fantasize.

• • •

About half of Americans talk with their partners about their sexual fantasies, according to ABC News.

• • •

When asked, "Who do you fantasize about?" by *Men's Health* magazine, 25% of men and 27.5% of women answered "a previous partner."

• • •

The survey showed that 22.7% of men and 19.2% of women fantasize about a friend.

• • •

And 20.5% of men and 26.7% of women fantasize about strangers.

• • •

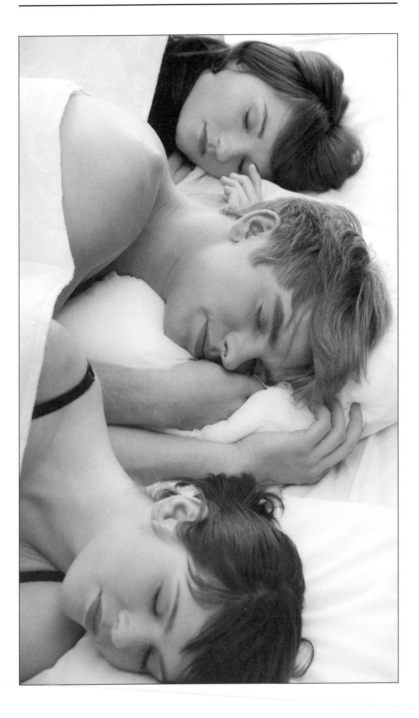

Amost 25% of men and 22.5% of women fantasize about celebrities and porn stars.

• • •

According to ABC News, 30% of Americans surveyed fantasize about cheating; 16% did it.

• • •

When asked by Kinsey Institute researchers, Americans tend to recollect a first sexual fantasy between the ages of 11-13 years old, with men recalling earlier fantasies than women.

• • •

According to WebMD, sex is better for your happiness than money. Increasing sex from once a month to once a week generates the happiness equal to getting an additional $50,000 in income for the average American. So in a very real way, changing the American Dream of being wealthy to being more sexually satisfied might be better for us all. Interestingly though, sex has a greater effect on the happiness of the highly educated than those with lower educational status. Going back to school never sounded so good . . . or at least get a library card and a willing partner.

Sexual daydreams can help women tune in to a sexual experience by helping to turn off the parts of the mind associated with stress and anxiety, according to *Women's Health* magazine.

• • •

A study in *The Journal of Sexual Medicine* found that if women ignore distractions, they can start to become aroused in just 30 seconds.

• • •

Nearly 70% of Americans admit to fantasizing about group sex at some point, according to RandomHistory.com, and more than 50% of those people actually follow through.

• • •

According to ABC News, 21% of Americans fantasize about a threesome and 10% of Americans fantasize about sex at work.

• • •

Just over 7% of men and 4.1% of women surveyed by *Men's Health* fantasize sexually about their coworkers.

• • •

According to the Trojan U.S. Sex Census, when asked where they would like to have sex but have not yet tried, 33% of men fantasize about sex on a plane and 26% of women fantasize about sex on a beach/sea.

• • •

According to the Kinsey Institute, sexual fantasies are healthy, occurring in people with the least sexual amount of sexual problems and least sexual dissatisfaction.

• • •

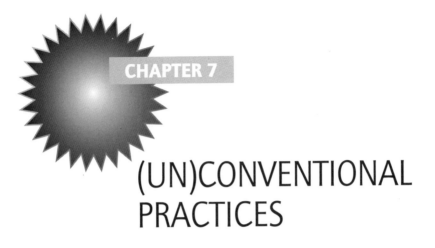

(UN)CONVENTIONAL PRACTICES

A grand sense of adventure and invention has always been a part of the American tradition—how else could one country have Lewis and Clark, Edison and Earhart, Armstrong and Jobs? The American personality includes creativity, experiment, and daring by nature—our very nation was called the Great Democratic Experiment. Americans continue this tradition daily and nightly, in their careers and in between the sheets. So how adventurous are we?

• • •

These are the habits that don't get talked about much, a look at the less conventional behavior of Americans and how comfortable we are with them. It's an examination of not just the fringes of society, but the odd little nooks and crannies in plain sight, and even how much normal people really enact some of their more risqué fantasies. There might be daredevils all around you, arranging a rendez-vous on the beach, in the parking lot, or the library. Even if you've never felt curious yourself, you've probably wondered who *has* felt curious. Who knows what secrets lay in drawers by the bed, or as edible drawers in the bed. How far will America go?

• • •

Newlyweds traditionally kiss at weddings because once upon a time kisses were used primarily to seal contracts— also why X's signify kisses in writing and a signature on contracts (OMG-Facts).

• • •

Thirty percent of participants in an Indiana University study don't consider oral sex to be sex. A number of older men do not even consider traditional vaginal intercourse to be sex. The number of people who consider vaginal intercourse to count as sex even drops by 6% when there is no ejaculation.

• • •

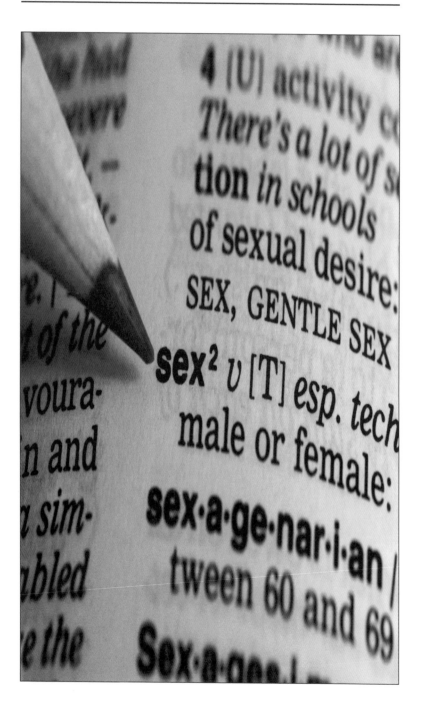

In a survey conducted by Harris Interactive, when asked how they personally define sex, given the choices vaginal, oral, and anal, more than 4% of both men and women chose "other."

• • •

According to a *Playboy* reader survey, 22% of men and 32% of women have tried some form of bondage during sex.

• • •

A study done by the Kinsey Institute found that 71% of heterosexual males, 11% of heterosexual females, and 12% of homosexual males prefer a dominant role when engaged in sexual bondage.

. . .

Almost 45% of men and 41.3% of women polled by *Men's Health* have used light bondage.

. . .

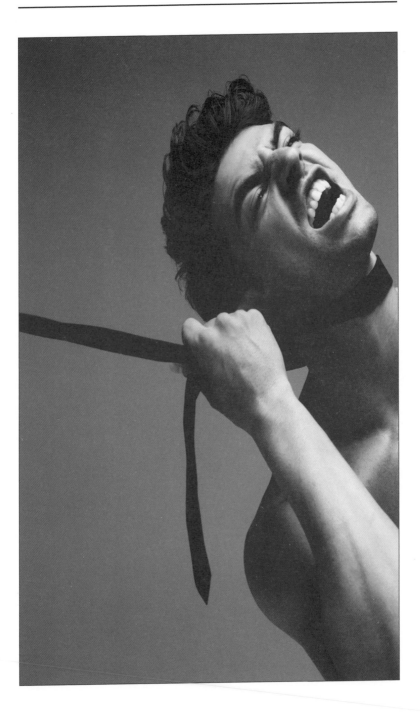

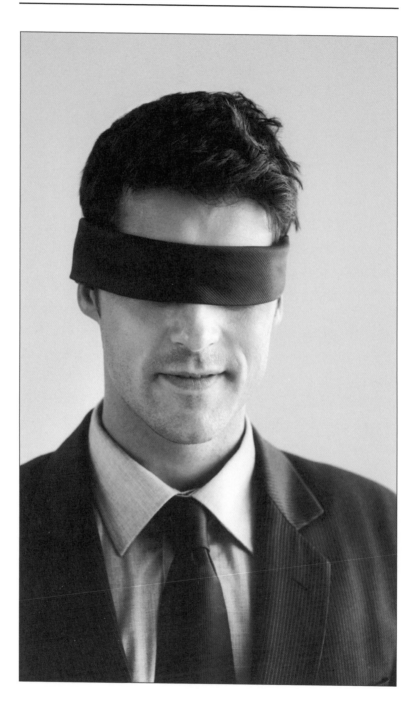

According to a Harris Interactive survey of Americans, 11% of men and 8% of women have used a sex toy.

. . .

Thirty-one percent of self-identifying liberal Americans polled by Harris Interactive have had sex with a foreigner. The survey also revealed that 38% of conservatives have posted a sex ad while in a relationship and that 46% of liberals and 26% of conservatives have had interracial sex.

. . .

Nearly 40% of men would love to have their sexual partner blindfold them, tie them up, or role-play, according to *Cosmo* magazine. Nineteen percent would enjoy spanking or anal touching.

. . .

According to a *Men's Health* magazine survey, 31.3% of men and 28.1% of women have used role playing.

. . .

Slightly more than 23 percent of men and 19% of women have videotaped sex.

• • •

More than half (15.3%) of male and 39% of female *Men's Health* readers have used sex toys.

• • •

According to the Kinsey Institute, BDSM stands for "Bondage, Discipline, Domination/Submission, Sadism/Masochism."

· · ·

Every year in San Francisco, some 400,000 people attend the Folsom Street Fair, an outdoor festival dedicated to the safer and more commercial aspect of sadomasochism, according to ABC news. The Fair claims to be the world's largest leather/fetish event, covering 13 city blocks. The 28th annual Folsom Street Fair will happen on September 23, 2012.

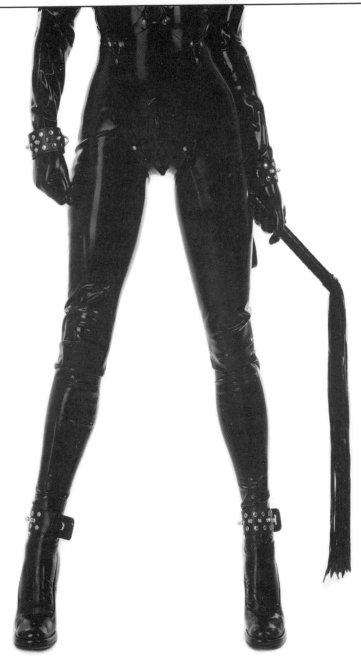

According to a survey conducted by the National Coalition for Sexual Freedom (NCS Freedom), 57% of respondents were out about their involvement in BDSM/Leather/Fetish practices, while 43% were not.

• • •

Out of the 3,058 American adults who responded to the NCS Freedom survey, 90.8% participate in bondage and discipline; 90% participate in dominance and submission; 80% in spanking; 76.8% in sadomasochism (S&M); 64.2% in leather; 60.1% in role-playing; 53.6% in exhibitionism; 52.2% in polyamory; 47.9% in voyeurism; 48.1% in cloth-

ing fetish; 44% in humiliation; 41.8% in fisting; 36% in wa-
tersports; 28.8% in body modification; 27.5% in medical
scenes; 18% in foot fetish; 12.9% in cross-dressing; and
14.5% participate in yet various other sexual exploits that
would be categorized under BDSM.

• • •

Almost 35% of respondents to the NCS Freedom survey
said that they've curtailed their use of the Internet for fear
of being judged or prosecuted.

• • •

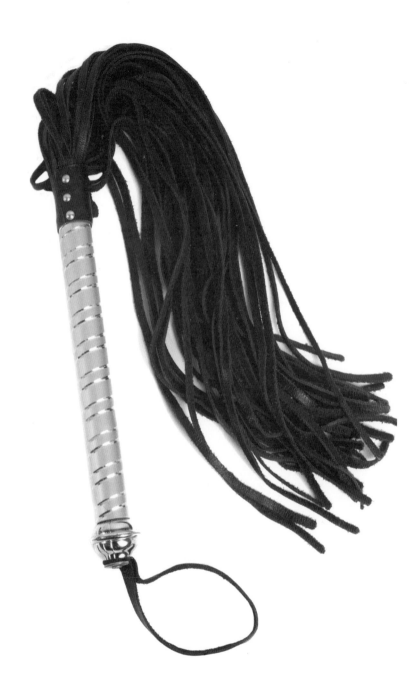

As for females, 36% of black women said they used a condom their last time, while 20% of white women claimed they did.

• • •

According to the National Survey of Sexual Health and Behavior, the older Americans become the less likely they are to use condoms, with the highest rate of usage being in the 14–17 range.

• • •

According to *Men's Health* magazine, only 9.5% of men and 8.8% of women reported having had a threesome.

• • •

More than 99% of women 15–44 who have ever had sex with a man have used at least one contraceptive method, according to the CDC. The leading method in 2008 was the oral contraceptive pill, with 10.7 million female users. The second most popular method was female sterilization, used by 10.3 million women.

• • •

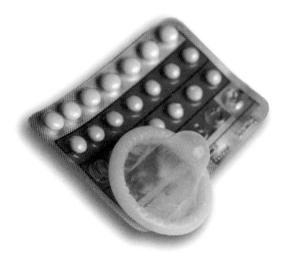

Almost 19% of the men and 14% of the women surveyed by *Men's Health* magazine claim to have had a threesome. For 50.3% of men and 49% of women, the demographics were two women and one man.

. . .

Just under 30% of women have been with two guys; 57.7% of men and 48.6% of women were not in a relationship with any of the other participants. Men were more likely to enjoy a threesome and be willing to do it again. On the other hand, 57.6% of women surveyed said they would never have a threesome.

• • •

According to ABC News 15% of men—and three in 10 single men age 30+—have paid for sex.

• • •

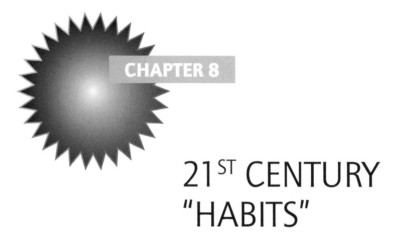

21ST CENTURY "HABITS"

It's a new era, and with interconnectedness changing our daily lives, it can't help but change the habits of intercourse. Not all that long ago, smart phones and social networks didn't mediate most of our relationships, but now they've changed the way people meet, flirt, and get intimate. Sharing has become a feature of our new social order, and twenty-first century technology permeates the possibilities.

. . .

With our laptops and computers, people of all ages and types are exploring what it means to be sexual and online. Thanks to the medium, passions have inflamed, marriages have been made, and politicians humiliated—all in new and exciting ways. It would be irresponsible to ignore the Internet's dangers—and there are more than a few. Meeting people can be unsafe and should be done with caution and through legitimate means. Sharing can quickly become a liability, as several former public figures can attest—everyone should be aware of the risks of sexting and pictures. This chapter looks at America's newly formed habits when it comes to our modern amenities—one last take on those questions who's doing what, when, and how. It's a guide to the sex habits of Americans as we step into the future, a new look on the land of (sexual) opportunity.

• • •

More than half of men surveyed by *Cosmo* magazine would love to videotape sex with their partner.

• • •

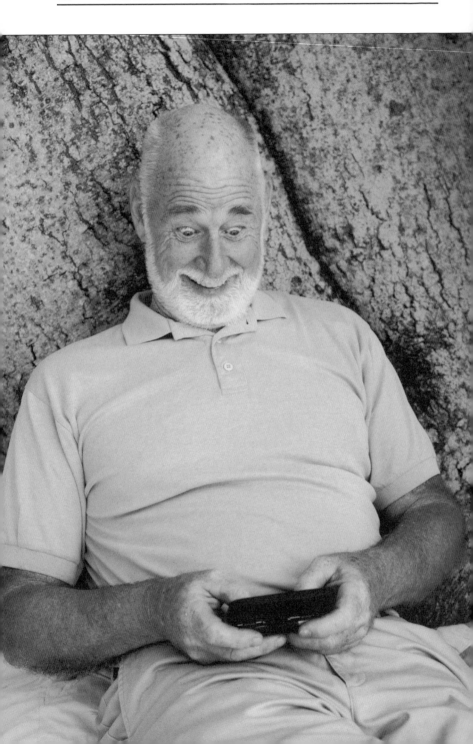

According to a *Men's Health* survey, 23.1% of American men and 19% of American women have videotaped sex.

. . .

According to a *Playboy* reader poll, 71% of women say they've tried "sexting" with a partner.

. . .

Almost half of men and 13% of women masturbate to online porn according to data from a Harris Interactive sex survey.

. . .

Nearly half of men, 45%, have visited a porn site in the past five years. Only 8% of women have done so, according to Harris Interactive.

. . .

A Harris sex survey showed that 32% of men and 4% of women have pornography stored on their computers.

• • •

Only 8% of men and 5% of women reported to Harris Interactive that they found their last sex partner online.

• • •

Sixteen percent of American adults have "sexted" someone on their phone. Another 16% have answered the phone
during sex, and 20% have participated in phone sex with a
partner, according to Harris Interactive.

• • •

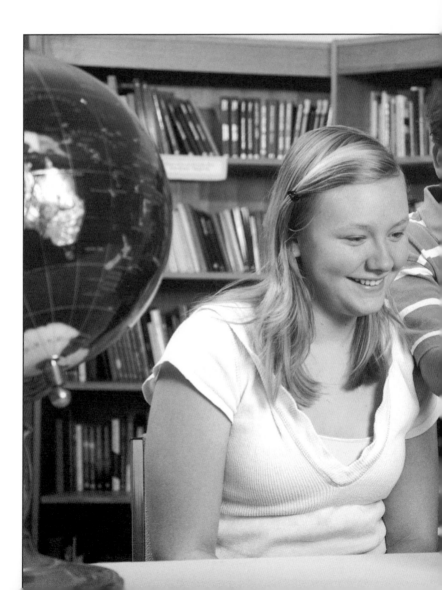

According to a Trojan condoms sex survey, 19% of Americans have engaged in "sexting" and 19% have had sex online.

. . .

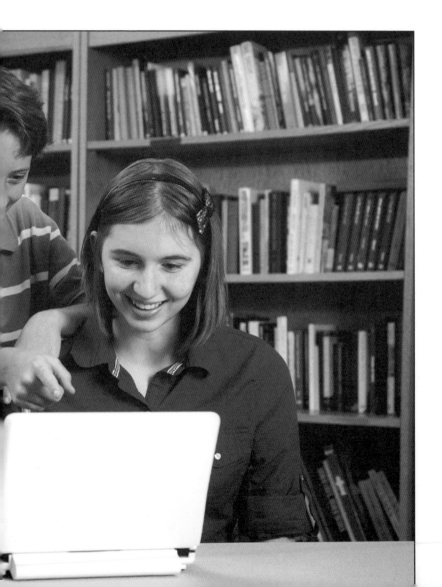

Of those surveyed by Trojan 18% have had sex with some-one they've met over the Internet.

• • •

Forty-three percent of women surveyed by *Playboy* maga-zine said they used an online dating site while already in a relationship.

• • •

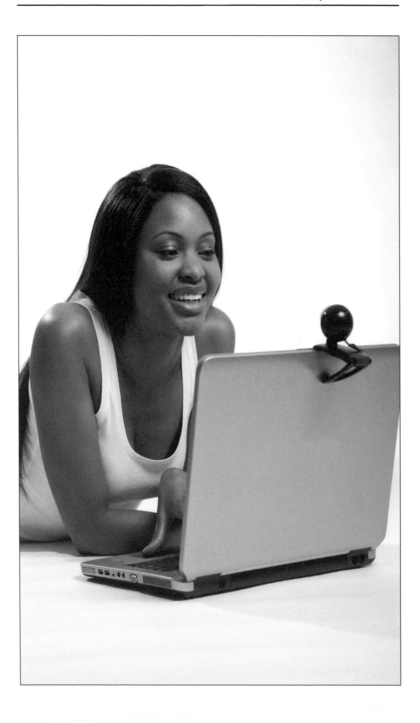

Just 10% of respondents have discussed sex on Facebook and/or Twitter, according to Trojan. Men were more likely to discuss their sex lives on social networks (15%) compared to the women (6%).

• • •

Slightly more than 40% of adolescent Internet users (10–17 years old), according to the Kinsey Institute, had been exposed to Internet pornography within the last year of being surveyed. A vast majority, 66%, claim those exposures to be unwanted.

• • •

According to *Cosmo Girl*, 22% of teen girls (13–19) have sent/posted sexually suggestive content of themselves; 18% of boys have done the same.

• • •

An estimated 87% of university students have had sex over webcam, instant messenger, or telephone according to BlazingGrace.com.

. . .

According to *Cosmo Girl*, 36% of young adult women and 31% of young adult men (20–16) are sending/posting sexually suggestive content of themselves.

. . .

Only 10% of Americans have discussed sex on Facebook and/or Twitter according to a survey by the makers of Trojan condoms.

• • •

Seventy-two percent of young adult women and 70% of young adult men tell *Cosmo Girl* that they send or post sexually suggestive content to be "fun or flirtatious." And 59% of young adult women say they've sent/posted sexually suggestive material just as a present for their boyfriend. In addition, 41% of young adult women and 51% of young adult men say they've sent such content simply in response to receiving it.

• • •

The fastest growing sex toy market, according to the *Examiner*, is American women over the age of 40.

• • •

Eighty percent of men and 94% of women have used a vibrator, according to a survey done by *Playboy*. Compare that their results from 1983 when the numbers were much lower: 32% of men and 49% of women had used a vibrator.

• • •

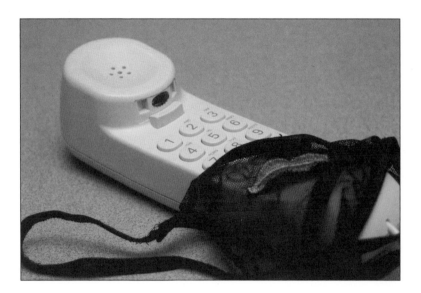

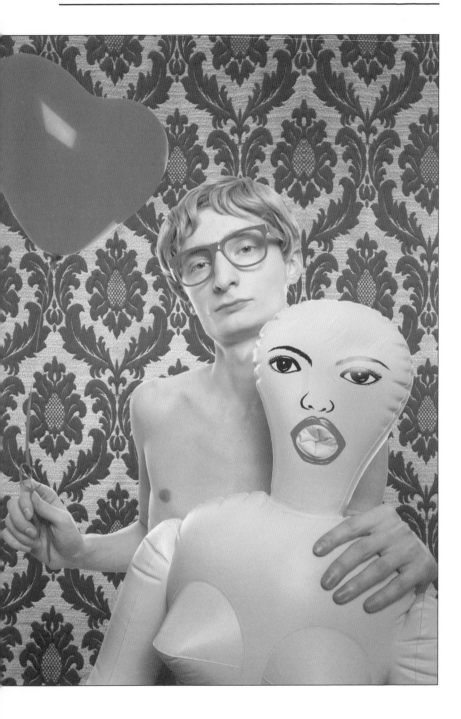

A life-size rubber doll developed by a New Jersey company is being dubbed "the world's first sex robot" according to an article in the *Huffington Post*. The doll is capable of engaging the owner with conversation rather than any lifelike movement.

• • •

Men make up two-thirds of users of pornographic Internet sites and account for 77% of online time, according to the Kinsey Institute.

• • •

One in every four dollars spent on the sex industry (movies, toys, phone sex) is spent by a woman, according to *Marie Claire.*

• • •

More than half of women reported to the Kinsey Institute that they've never download sexual material.

• • •

The vibrator was initially developed as a medicinal treatment for female "hysteria" during the nineteenth century, according to SheKnows.com.

• • •

According to the *Examiner*, most sex toy owners are in a relationship and not alone despite popular perception.

• • •

The sale of sex toys and vibrators is banned in Alabama and Mississippi. Texas overturned the ban as recently as 2008, according to Fox News.

· · ·

Seventeen percent of American women are using online pornography for sexual gratification according to *Marie Claire*.

· · ·

Anal bleaching has gained a lot of popularity in recent years, according to *Marie Claire*, with creams being available for purchase as easily as cough drops.

· · ·

Butt Botox, vaginal rejuvenation, labia correction, clitoral "unhooding," g-spot enhancement, and pelvic muscle tightening are all procedures more readily available and common in modern times, according to *Marie Claire* magazine.

• • •

According to *Glamour* magazine, a racy new product currently available to satisfy multiple needs of the modern woman is the "Little Rooster alarm clock." Part vibrator, part alarm clock, the wide flat head rests against a woman's pubic bone and its vibrating leg rests against the clitoris and labia to stimulate awakening.

According to the *LA Times* magazine, in America, 11,000 adult films are produced each year in Hollywood—more than 20 times the mainstream movie production.

• • •

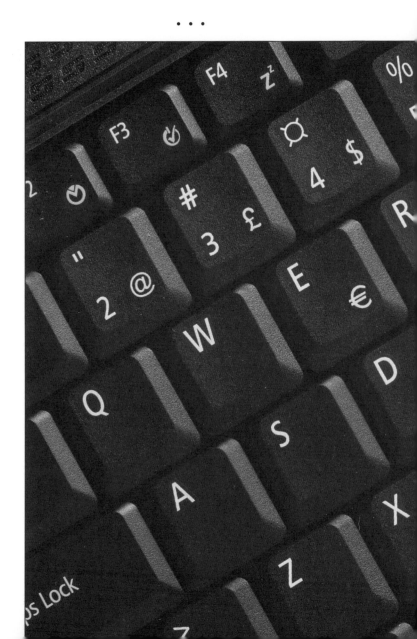

Thirty percent of Americans use sexually explicit videos to enhance their sex lives, according to ABC News.

. . .

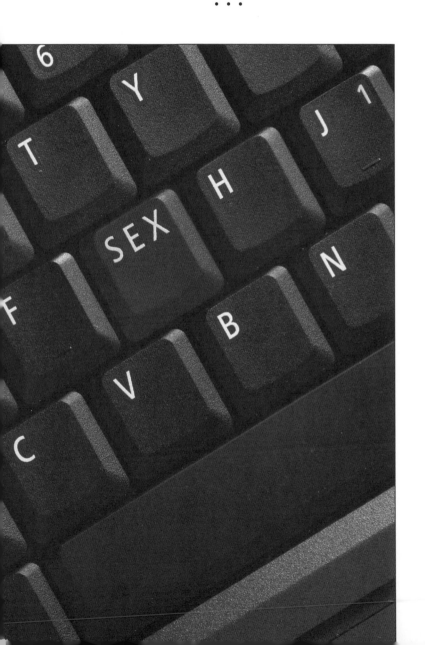

According to TechCrunch.com, 260 new porn sites go on-line daily.

• • •

Twelve percent of all websites and 8% of all emails are pornographic, according to data collected by United Families International.

• • •

According to United Families International, Utah has the country's highest online porn subscription rate per thousand home broadband users: 5.47.

• • •

One in five Americans surveyed by ABC news—around 40 million people—say they've looked at porn online.

• • •

Elmhurst, IL is the number one city in the U.S. to search the Internet for terms such as "Sex," "Porn," and "XXX," according to Family Safe Media's pornography statistics.

• • •

The Kinsey Institute estimates more than half of all online spending to be sexual in nature.

• • •

According to Family Safe Media, $3, 075.64 is being spent on pornography every second.

• • •